Essential Oils 101

Essential Oils Guide For Beginners

Table of Contents

Introduction

I want to thank you and congratulate you for downloading the book, *"Essential Oils 101: Essential Oils Guide for Beginners"*.

This book contains proven steps and strategies on how:

- To enjoy the full benefits of using essential oils, and why you should give up common beliefs about essential oils;
- To choose only pure and high quality oils and how to distinguish them from other oils
- To choose good essential oils even as a beginner
- You can enjoy the use of essential oils and have no worries regarding possible adverse effects and complications
- To avail safer and economical natural remedy done at the comfort of your home

Use this book as your handy reference in getting started with essential oils. The content is basic and meant even for those who are just about to start their journey of benefiting from the use of essential oils.

Understand, however, that the content of this book is not meant to substitute professional advice and recommendation from your health expert. It is meant to increase your knowledge and understanding to help you with your prudent decisions.

Thanks again for downloading this book. I hope you enjoy it!

Chapter 1:

Discarding Prevailing Essential Oil Myths

Beginners are prone to holding on to their common beliefs.

If you wish to get the most from essential oils, you should be able to differentiate facts from wrong information and say-so.

Essential oils as a topic, is very wide in range. Because of this, a lot of information is known and spread about these oils which sometimes lead to misinformation.

To avail of the full benefits you can get from essential oils, don't let these ten big myths fool you.

Therapeutic Grade

Myth #1: All essential oils you can find in the market are therapeutic grade.

That's just plain wrong. Not all available oils are 100% pure and high quality essential oils. An essential oil can be 100% pure but low quality.

Tampering with purity and quality is what makes some of the oils non-therapeutic grade.

What you can rely on is the amount of aromatic compounds found in the oil. The more the aromatic compounds kept and preserved within the oil, the better and the closer it is to therapeutic grade.

It is not surprising that many beginners are victims of this myth though. For one thing, it is difficult to determine if essential oils are genuinely therapeutic. The reason is the absence of standards.

Companies and manufacturers create their own standards, and therapeutic grade, having no concrete or definite meaning because of the absence of standards, is just a term companies and manufacturers use for promotion of their product.

The thing is, in the absence of standards, manufacturers follow their own standards. There are a lot of "standards" used in considering which oils are therapeutic grade.

The standards set may be different from one company to another.

There are also a lot of factors considered when creating standards for therapeutic grade oil. These include the physical and environmental factors.

The physical factors include looking at the process of bottling, harvesting, and distilling the plant. The environmental factors include looking at the conditions and environment of the place where the plant was cultivated.

These may or may not include third party quality control. For an essential oil to be of therapeutic grade, it has to be: (1) 100% pure, and (2) high quality.

Purity & Quality

Myth #2: Pure essential oils are high quality.

When it comes to essential oils, purity and quality are not one and the same.

Essential oils can be 100% pure, but it can also be of low quality. If they are adulterated or not pure, it follows that they are low quality.

Meanwhile, high quality essential oils are always 100% pure.

Essential oils undergo a process in order to be called high quality.

It takes time and money to be able to come up with the correct chemical proportions of the oil that will have a corresponding and certain effect on the body.

One way to know if the oils are high quality is to look at the aromatic compounds left in the oil. The more aromatic compounds preserved within the oil, the better.

Here are some of the factors that affect the purity of the oil:

- Combination of the same type of oil, e.g. lavender oil, but of different quality. For instance, one is high quality lavender oil, and the other is low quality lavender oil.
- Combination of two to several different types of oil, e.g. lavender oil and chamomile, not all of which are high quality.
- Adding other substances to the oil, either natural substances or artificial substances.
- Adding base oils, e.g. olive oil, to the essential oil and passing the mixture as pure essential oil.

Factors that affect the quality of the oil:

The country where the essential oil came from
The climate in that country
Condition of the Soil and Rainfall
Altitude
The use of chemicals and pesticides
The method by which the plant was grown and harvested
Difficulty in distinguishing between plant varieties and species
The gap between harvest time and processing time
The type of oil extraction
The condition of the plant prior to the extraction
Packaging conditions
Storage conditions
Containers of the oil
Delivery handling
Chemical degradation (Oxidation, Exposure to light, Heat)

Shelf Life

Myth #3: Essential oils last forever.

Once opened, the shelf life of most essential oils last for 2 or more years.

Yes, essential oils may last for a long time but they do not remain good for use forever. Essential oils undergo chemical degradation through time. It may be because of exposure to light or oxidation. Some oils however, get better through time to a certain point. Some of these are patchouli, assertive, and sandalwood.

High sesquiterpene alcohol oils which are heavier are typically the ones that become better through time. Most essential oils, however, degrade chemically with time. Examples of these are citrus and blue oils.

The high concentration of limonene in citrus oils is what causes it to oxidize fast when compared to other oils. The formation of limonene oxide in citrus oils can change the odor of the oil completely.

Because of this, citrus oils, as much as possible, are only good for use within a year or so.

Essential Oils During Biblical Times

Myth #4: Essential oils existed during the biblical times.

Essential oils undergo the process of distillation which did not yet exist during the biblical times.

Aromatic substances were used during the biblical times but these aromatic substances are different from what we call essential oils in the present.

The aromatic materials used during the biblical times were just plants and herbs soaked in pressed oil and animal fats.

The process of distillation was created only in the 10th century and it could not have existed during the biblical times. Do not confuse aromatic substances during the biblical times with what we call today as essential oils.

Detox

Myth #5: Essential oils are natural so its effects are always good.

If an essential oil gives you a rash or a burn, it does not mean that your body is detoxifying.

A lot of people believe that if something is natural, its effects are always good.

This is the reason why even when the initial effect of rubbing an essential oil on their body is a rash or a burn, they refuse to believe that its a negative effect and rather, tell themselves that it is just their body detoxifying.

Detoxifying is a process that removes a harmful or poisonous substance such as alcohol or drugs from the body. When using essential oils, detoxifying is not possible because no substance is removed from the body.

Instead, something new is added to the body. If you experience a bad reaction when rubbing a certain essential oil to your body, it does not mean that your body is just detoxifying.

It means that it is irritating your skin and you should stop the use of this essential oil as soon as possible.

Chapter 2:

Facts You Should Know about Essential Oil

Your best weapon against myths and fallacies are facts.

The effects and certain reactions of essential oils are not the same for all people which is a big reason why you should not believe say so and base your preferences to the experience of other people.

Knowing and understanding factual information about essential oils will allow you to enjoy the full benefits.

Essential Oils vs. Fragrance Oils

Beginners and even non-beginners often confuse essential oils with fragrance oils and vice versa. The reason for this confusion is because of the scent.

As such, most people use both oils for almost the same purposes.

It should be known that essential oils come from substances that naturally occur from different parts of plants like the flowers, leaves, resin, wood, bark, stem and fruits. Essential oils undergo the process of distillation, which takes time and money.

The chemicals that occur naturally in essential oils are about 50 to 500 in number and can have varying effects. Fragrance oils, on the other hand, do not use natural substances.

Fragrance oils use artificial substances to come up with artificial fragrances. These oils also do not undergo the process of distillation, as essential oils do, which makes these oils less expensive.

Essential oils also have different uses from fragrance oils. Essential oils are used to improve the physical, mental, and emotional health of a person.

It may relieve pain, inflammation, or improve a person's mood. Fragrance oils, on the other hand, are used to make artificial scents for perfumes, soaps, and candles.

The term essential oils and fragrance oils are two terms that are commonly used interchangeably.

However, essential oils and fragrance oils are two different things. They differ in their chemical composition and they have different properties. The following table illustrates major differences between the two.

Category	Essential Oils	Fragrance Oils
Purpose/Use	Aromatherapy, Natural Remedy, Healing Purposes(Physical, Mental, and Emotional)	Air Freshener, Perfume Ingredient, Cosmetic Purposes, Artificial scent for soaps and candles
Composition	Natural (Extracted from Plants), Scent has shorter duration	Synthetic, Artificial Scent lasts longer
Price	Price fluctuates, but it is usually more expensive than fragrance oils	Steady price and less expensive than essential oils

Why Quality & Purity Matter

In choosing essential oils, quality and purity are crucial. The reasons are as follows:

- Purity alone is not enough. A pure essential oil can be of low quality and cause negative reactions from the body. The belief that untouched essential oils will have better therapeutic effects is not true. One example is the use of pure and unbuffered aspirin. Using this can cause a stomachache and can even lead to stomach ulcers.
- Purity and quality enable you to distinguish therapeutic grade essential oils. Only therapeutic grade oils, which are both high quality and pure, are with the correct chemical proportions which will have a certain effect on the body. Essential oils that are not both high quality and 100% pure may have chemical proportions which can cause unpredictable effects on the body.
- You'll be able to differentiate it from other types such as fragrance oils using purity and quality as gauge. Fragrance oils use artificial substances and are made for different purposes. Confusing fragrance oils with essential oils may lead to the wrong usage of these oils which can cause negative reactions.
- Purity and quality is what will make essential oils effective for healing purposes. Only the correct chemical proportions in an oil can make it effective for healing purposes. Those who practice holistic medicine recognize the necessity and importance of using only 100% pure essential oils with high quality.
- Results depend so much on the quality and purity of the oils. Using tampered or adulterated oils for therapeutic purposes will only bring no results at best. These oils may cause unpredictable reactions from the body. At worst, such oils may trigger adverse reactions and complications ranging from mild to severe to life-threatening.

High Concentration & Dilution

It is not advisable to use essential oils undiluted. In fact, you must never use it without diluting, especially if you are going to use it on your dog or your baby. This is because essential oils are highly concentrated.

There are, however, essential oils that are recognized generally to be safe for undiluted use. Rose geranium, tea tree, sandalwood, and lavender are acknowledged as safe to use sparingly.

Using undiluted oils should be with precaution and under the guidance of an aromatherapy practitioner who is experienced.

Using essential oils undiluted may cause irritation of the skin and sensitization. There have been cases where the undiluted use of essential oils has caused stinging and burning sensations upon application.

In worse cases, second degree burns were experienced.

Reactions of sensitization are also common. But the reactions differ depending on the amount and type of essential oil used and the chemistry of the skin.

Once a person develops sensitization to a certain type of essential oil, that person will remain sensitized to that essential oil even when diluted.

Also, never use undiluted essential oils on your baby. The skin of babies is much thinner and sensitive when compared to adults and therefore, are much more prone to irritation and sensitization.

When using essential oils on babies, only half of the required amount in the recipe is needed.

Dilution is a necessary process with essential oils. It makes the oil safe for use. Dilution is a process where essential oils are combined with carrier oils or real oils. You do not use essential oils as they are.

You need to dilute the oil before you can use it safely for its benefits. Otherwise, the undiluted essential oils may cause irritations on your skin. Examples of carrier oils are alcohols, butters, and waxes.

How to Dilute

The process of dilution is simple. You mix essential oils with carrier oils or real oils. However, the amount to add varies depending on how you wish to use your diluted essential oil. The following table can serve as your quick reference:

.25% dilution	1 drop of essential oil add to 4 teaspoons of carrier oil	Suitable for children, although it is best to avoid using essential oils for children. Consult your physician before using the diluted solution.
1% dilution	1 drop of essential oil add to 1 teaspoon of carrier oil	For the elderly, persons with weak or compromised immune system, persons who have sensitive skin, persons who suffer from major health issues
2% dilution	2 drops of essential oil add to 1 teaspoon of carrier oil	Most of the adults and in most situations. Usually, this is the best dilution for skin care purposes.
3% dilution	3 drops of essential oil add to 1 teaspoon of carrier oil	For adults who need only temporary solution for short-term health issues.

Carrier Oils

Since dilution is a necessary process for the safe use of essential oils, carrier oils are needed. Carrier oils come from a plant's fatty portion like its kernel, seeds, or nuts.

The purpose of carrier oils is the reason for its name. A carrier oil carries an essential oil so it can be applied safely on the skin. Carrier oils can affect the aroma, color, and overall properties of an essential oil.

Depending on the benefits wanted, the type of carrier oil used varies. Here are some of the common carrier oils to mix with essential oils:

Virgin (Pure) Coconut Oil	Contains anti-microbial, anti-fungal, antioxidant and antibacterial properties that is most suitable for skin care and moisturizing, hair care, diaper rash, and to treat dry lips. It is also a good massage oil. If you wish to use essential oils for your dog, then coconut oil is perhaps the best carrier oil. The benefits of this oil are primarily brought by the presence of caprylic acid, capric acid, and lauric acid which is also have excellent antibacterial properties
Almond Oil	This is a multi-purpose carrier oil. It has vitamins E, B, and A that is good for the skin. It helps moisturize the skin and can also cure dry skin. Almond oil can soothe inflammations and irritations. It is the most suitable for getting rid of dark circles. Removing make-up using almond oil is very ideal. It can also reduce hair fall and help get rid of split ends. It works well with spicy essential oils such as cinnamon. It is also the base oil that is most suitable for massage therapy that relieves joint and muscle pains.
Jojoba Oil	If you are looking for a stable carries that will not go rancid, this one is it. The skin absorbs this oil very well and because of this, it is nice to use as skin moisturizer and facial cleanser. It nourishes the scalp and softens the hair which makes it suitable for hair care. It can minimize the appearance of scars and stretch marks. Jojoba oil contains iodine which can prevent blackheads, pimples, and breakouts. It can also promote hair growth. Jojoba oil is most suitable for skin care and hair care treatment.

Olive Oil	This is an all-purpose carrier oil suitable for cooking, skin care, or herbal remedy. It contains properties that heal and disinfect.
	Olive oil contains the antioxidants polyphenols, vitamin E, and phytosterols which help fight the signs of aging. It helps in the gentle exfoliation of the skin because of its ability to remove dead skin cells.
	Olive oil can also moisturize the skin, prevent clogging of pores, strengthen the nails, and hydrate the skin around the eyes.
Avocado Oil	Avocado oil is the carrier oil that is rich in essential fatty acids as well as Vitamins A, D, E, and K. It treats skin problems like itchiness, eczema and psoriasis.
	It can stimulate and increase collage production which fights away the signs of aging. Vitamins A, D, and E found in this oil can also cure skin that is damaged from the sun.
	Potassium and lecithin can also be found in the oil which is good for the skin and the hair. Perform a skin test first before using this oil since it is not suitable for people who are allergic to latex. Avoid this if you will use the mixture to your dog.
Borage Seed Oil	This oil is rich in GLA (gamma linolenic acid) which is known to relieve dry and sensitive skin.
	It can also help cure redness and skin inflammations. Skin disorders like dermatitis and eczema can be cured by this oil.
	Borage Seed Oil is most suitable for skin care treatment.
Apricot Kernel Oil	Apricot kernel oil can be used in cooking, skin care and hair care.
	This oil is non-irritant which means that it is suitable for sensitive skin.

	It can help make the skin smooth and it has properties that can fight the signs of aging. It is a good massage oil because it easily makes the skin smooth and soft and once absorbed, the skin remains moisturized for a long time.
	It has an antiseptic property which can minimize infection in cuts and open wounds. This oil also has a lot of nutrients in it like Vitamin E which is very suitable for hair care.
Camellia Seed Oil	Camellia seed oil, also known as tea oil, come from the plants which are used to make tea.
	It is good for skin care, hair care, and can also be used in cooking. This oil has a number of therapeutic properties which include antioxidant, emollient, cicatrizant, and analgesic.
	Antioxidant properties of this oil strongly resists rancidity. Emollient properties promote skin moisturizing. Cicatrizant helps cure wounds faster. Analgesic properties of the oil help relieve pain.
	The oil is also a good emulsifying agent which is good to find in cosmetic products. Camellia seed oil is very light and is best suited for skin and hair care.
Sesame Oil	This oil has Vitamin E and emollient properties which is good for skin moisturizing.
	Sesame oil has the micro nutrient sesamol which can help fight the signs of aging such as wrinkles and fine lines. It has antioxidant properties that protects the skin from harmful UV rays.
	Though it is heavier than the other oils, sesame oil can also be used as a massage oil and through the skin, it can detoxify the body. This oil is also good for promoting hair growth and treating damaged hair.
Grapeseed Oil	Grapeseed oil is a very light oil. It has properties like anti-inflammatory and antioxidant properties which

	makes it suitable for treating acne and other skin conditions or irritations. This oil contains oligomeric procyanidin, a flavonoid which is a very good antioxidant. This helps protect the body from free radicals which may cause cellular damage. Because of its lightness, it is easily absorbed by the skin which makes it a good massage oil and moisturizer. Grape seed oil is most suitable for skin care.
Peanut oil	This oil has polyphenol antioxidants which help fight free radicals. It has properties which help cure acne, moisturize skin, and get rid of dandruff. Peanut oil also contains resveratrol which can help lower blood pressure. This oil is a good massage oil and can also be used in cooking.
Wheatgerm Oil	Wheatgerm oil is rich in vitamin E which gives it its antioxidant properties. Because of this, it is commonly used to increase the shelf life of other carrier oils. This oil is also suitable for massage when mixed with other oils as it helps in the circulation of the blood and cell formation. Wheatgerm oil is most suitable for skin care purposes.

Chapter 3:

The Safest Essential Oils for Beginners

While essential oils are generally safe to use, some are safer than the others. For beginners, you are better off starting your experience with these essential oils.

Lavender

Lavender is the safest among essential oils for adults. It is the best oil to start your experience with aromatherapy. Pure lavender oil has several therapeutic benefits and helps with the following conditions:

- Restlessness
- Depression
- Stress and anxiety
- Nervousness
- Insomnia
- Upset stomach
- Appetite loss
- Nausea
- Vomiting
- Indigestion
- Urine flow
- Flatulence
- Respiratory disorders
- Circulation of blood
- Migraine
- Headaches

- Wounds and burns
- Psoriasis
- Eczema
- Hair loss
- Toothache
- Joint and muscle pains
- Sores
- Acne

It is also effective as:

- Mosquito repellent
- Flea bites
- Flea and tick repellent

Evidence is strong for the following conditions:

- Alopecia areata or hair loss – combined with other essential oils, lavender promotes hair growth up to 44% under a 7-month hair and scalp treatment. According to a study, 40% of the people who were suffering from hair loss experienced positive results when lavender oil was applied on their scalp regularly. This is because of the properties of lavender oil which stimulates the circulation of blood. Because lavender is regenerative, it can be found in a lot of solutions and formulas that promote hair growth.
- The best oils to combine with lavender for this purpose are the following: rosemary, thyme, and cedar wood.
- Pain associated with child delivery – inhaling diluted solution of lavender essential oils after child delivery via caesarian section reduces pain significantly. A massage using lavender oil is also a good way to help ease the pain and relax during labor. This is because of the chemicals and analgesic properties that are contained within the lavender essential oil which helps relieve the pain.
- Grapeseed oil is a good carrier oil to combine with lavender for this purpose.
- Canker sores – are painful sores in your mouth, usually at your gum base. Lavender essential oil contains anti-

inflammatory properties that may help cure canker sores. Applying diluted lavender essential oil on the affected area speeds up healing and relieves the pain and swelling.

Chamomile

Chamomile is a gentle yet powerful essential oil. It has a lot of therapeutic properties which include:

- Anti-inflammatory
- Antiseptic
- Antioxidant
- Analgesic
- Antibiotic
- Digestive tonic
- Sedative
- Antidepressant
- Hepatic
- Antipyretic
- Vermifuge
- Carminative
- Tonic

German Chamomile

This essential oil contains a compound called chamazulene which gives it its blue color. This compound is known to help the body's needs in fighting irritation. German chamomile properties can help treat the following conditions:

- Wounds and cuts
- Irritation from colds
- Flatulence
- Colic
- Insomnia
- Allergies
- Gum and skin inflammation
- Boils

- Sores
- Abscess
- Eczema
- Psoriasis
- Diaper rash
- Chickenpox
- Arthritis
- Dysmenorrhea
- Headache
- Stress

Roman Chamomile

Roman chamomile is an essential oil that is safe to use even for babies as long as it is well diluted. This oil is known for its good anti-inflammatory properties.

Compared to German chamomile, this oil works better in relieving pain and stress. Roman chamomile properties can help treat the following conditions:

- Sleeping difficulties such as insomnia
- Menstrual pain
- Headache
- Nausea
- Stress and anxiety
- Inflamed joints
- Wounds
- Allergies
- Boils
- Abscess
- Insect bites
- Sprains
- Cuts
- Sores

The following are other oils that blend well with Chamomile: lavender, rose, citrus oils, and geranium.

Lemon

Lemons are rich in vitamins and also help in the process of digestion. This essential oil is popular for its anti-bacterial properties.

Its other properties are antiseptic, anti-fungal, carminative, calming, and astringent properties.

According to a study, lemon possesses the best anti-microbial properties among all the essential oils. People use it as part of their treatment for infections and wounds. Other benefits include the following:

- Weight loss
- Help melt belly fat
- Strengthens the immune system
- Natural antibiotic for
  - Colds
  - Bronchitis
  - Throat infections
  - Flu
- Relieves tension and anxiety
- Relieves stress
- Headaches and migraines
- Improves mental health
- Increases focus and concentration
- Works as an anti-aging agent
- Flushes out toxic substances
- Stops bleeding
- Helps treat asthma
- Treats mouth ulcers, gum problems such as gingivitis
- Can get rid of warts
- Helps clear the skin from acne, boils, and spots
- Hair care
- Promotes hair growth
- Can help remedy discolored skin
- Can remove foul odors and disinfect at the same time

If you use lemon oil as a mouth rinse, it is always best to follow up with pure water. This is to protect your teeth against potential enamel erosion. Further, when you apply the diluted oil on your skin, make sure to avoid direct exposure to sunlight.

Lemon Oil Recipe

Here's a quick recipe to create your lemon essential oil:

Ingredients:

- 2 medium-sized lemons
- 1.2 cup of pure (virgin) olive oil

Procedure:

Zest the lemons.

In a saucepan over low heat, mix your lemon zest and olive oil.

Cook slowly up to 10 minutes. Remove from heat and let the oil cool.

Chapter 4:

Basic Methods of Using Essential Oils

In using essential oils, your goal should always be to use it safely. Understand that each essential oil has its own uses, and you can't use all of them in identical ways. Using essential oils for the wrong purposes may result to negative reactions from the body. Another important thing to follow when using essential oils: always start with less. This is especially applicable to testing if you are not allergic to the certain essential oil you are about to use.

Here are the basic methods of using essential oils safely.

Aromatic Use

Perhaps the most popular use of essential oils is in aromatherapy. This is because these oils emit scents that can calm the mind and body and help you to rest and relax. They are also known for their healing properties.

Benefits of using essential oils for aromatherapy include the following:

- Promotes rest and relaxation
- Improves mood and disposition
- Reduces stress
- Strengthens the immune system
- Improves blood circulation
- Nurtures the respiratory system
- Normalize hormone levels
- Aids in digestion
- Eases pain

The best side effect of essential oils is that it removes the toxins and other impurities in the air that you breathe. It minimizes your risks of airborne diseases.

To use essential oils for aromatherapy, you have the following options:

- Diffusing the scent in the air – use a good diffuser that will allow the molecules of the oil to linger in the air without affecting its structure. The diffuser should use room temperature or cool air.
- Direct or indirect inhalation – with about 5 inches away from your nose, you can inhale the scent of the oil directly from the bottle. You can also add one or two drops to a clean cloth or cotton ball for indirect inhalation. For safety purposes, though, it is always recommended to dilute the oil before inhalation.
- Steam inhalation – you can use certain oils, such as eucalyptus, for hot water steam inhalation. Remember to keep a safe distance away from the steam heat to prevent burns. Use hot water and not boiling water. Steam inhalation is often used to improve respiratory conditions.
- Massage – you can use one or more essential oils depending on your desired effect. Dilute the essential oils by only adding three to five drops of the oil on 10 ml carrier oil. Jojoba or other carrier oils can be used.
- Skin Care – for 30 ml of carrier oil, one drop of essential oil can be added. Essential oils like Geranium and Tea Tree are good oils to use as they moisturize the skin and prevent acne.
- Foot bath – you can use three to four drops of your chosen essential oil in a foot bath. The oils Rosemary, Peppermint, and Lavender are a good combination for a foot bath. Other essential oils that are comforting can also be used.
- Bath – you can use warm water with properly diluted essential oils in your bath. Essential oils with relaxing aromas such as Sandalwood, Lavender, and Roman Chamomile are recommended. You can mix six to eight drops of essential oil with warm water. For safety purposes,

make sure that you do not add more than eight drops of essential oil, especially when you are using multiple oils.

Topical Use

The process is simple, but needs a little more care and caution. Topical use involves applying the oil on the skin or the affected area. Keep in mind that some oils are not suitable for topical application. Perform a skin test to see your reaction to the oil before proceeding with its topical use.

Before applying the oil topically, be sure to dilute it. Refer to Chapter 2, How to Dilute for your easy reference. Do not worry about the concentration, as dilution oil will not affect the oil's effectiveness and value. Besides, dilution improves the absorption of oil by your skin. It also makes the essential oil safer to use.

Here are some of the best ways to use essential oils topically:

- Massage Therapy – 100% pure and high quality essential oils contain therapeutic properties. Massage is a popular remedy to ease muscle tension, get rid of stress, and relieve or reduce muscle and joint pain.

  Massaging with essential oils has the following benefits:

  o Improves digestive functions and prevent disorders
  o Eases pain during menstruation
  o Blood pressure control depending on essential oils used
  o Removes toxins
  o General reliever for headaches, nerve pain, and temporomandibular (TMJ) pain
  o Relaxes stressed muscles
  o Supports nervous system
  o Boosts immune system
  o Improves texture of skin
  o Treats insomnia associated with stress and anxiety
  o Works as a natural remedy for the following conditions: myofascial pain syndrome, strains and injuries
  o Draws positive feelings

Be sure to follow the safety precautions when massaging with essential oils. Know the risks of massage as well as the safety guidelines for the use of essential oils.

- Hot or Cold Compress – Hot or cold compress is a non-invasive therapy for pain relief. It is most effective in relieving muscle or joint pain especially when performing first aid. You apply hot compress for recurring or chronic pain, and cold compress for pain associated with sports injuries such as sprains, bumps, bruises, and strains.

In using essential oil for hot compress, never commit the mistake of heating the oil. Instead, pour a few drops of the essential oil on a clean towel or cloth, and wrap it in bottle filled with hot (not boiling) water.

To use for cold compress, soak your clean towel or cloth in cold water with a few drops of the oil. Place the towel or cloth over the affected area.

Precautions

When using essential oils for topical applications, observe the following precautions:

- Perform a skin test prior to the application. No matter how gentle the oil is, your skin may react differently to it. A skin test can save you from adverse effects.
- Follow the basic principle of "less is more" with essential oils. Always dilute your essential oil irrespective of how safe or mild the oil is.
- Always use 100% pure and high quality essential oil. Using adulterated or tampered oils can only result to adverse effects.

Internal Consumption

Although this method has the most profound effects, you have to be extra careful when using essential oils for internal consumption.

Not all oils are suitable to be taken internally. As much as you can, avoid internal consumption of oils for the following reasons:

- Much attention, care, and caution should go to choosing the essential oil to use. There are no standards by which you can pinpoint what oils are therapeutic and what oils are not. If this is a difficulty for you, best that you avoid ingesting essential oils.
- Even experts at using essential oils would not recommend internal consumption. The only exception is when your health practitioner, with adequate training on the use of essential oils, would recommend and guide you as you with the internal use of the oils.

Here are some of the ways to use essential oils for internal consumption:

- Mix with Water or Honey – you can use essential oils to add flavor to your water. For a glass of water, one drop of oil would be enough. Adding a drop of oil to every 5 ml of honey can also be done. The essential oils peppermint and lemon is suitable for this use.
- Freshen breath – you can use the essential oil peppermint to freshen your breath. One drop of this oil on your tongue will be enough to kill the bacteria to causes bad breath.
- Cooking – essential oils can add good flavors to your food. The heat used in cooking may remove a few of the healing properties of the essential oil but the flavor of the food will be enhanced by these oils. Lemon, for example, can be added to lemonade and this can lessen the sugar content of the drink.

Precautions

Observe the following precautions when using essential oils for ingestion:

Start with the lowest amount possible. This is because your liver has a tolerance limit for essential oils. If you need to follow a certain amount, break it down into frequency.

Never attempt to take essential oils internally without consulting your health practitioner. Guidance of an expert is necessary and critical to ensure safety of use. Otherwise, you run the risks of serious adverse effects and complications.

If you have high blood pressure or epilepsy, it is best to avoid using essential oils for internal consumption. You should see your doctor first before taking in any essential oil.

Using essential oils for internal consumption is not advisable for children under six years of age. Children may be more sensitive to these essential oils and their bodies may respond to these oils differently compared to adults.

Miscellaneous Applications For Your Home

Essential oils are versatile natural remedy not only for you and your family including your dog, but also for your home. Here's how your home can benefit from its use:

Natural Air Freshener – through diffusion, your home can smell refreshingly good with your preferred essential oil. What's more, the oil has the ability to kill pathogens that can cause airborne diseases.

Fabric Freshener – you just need 10 drops of essential oil added to 2 cups of water with a tablespoon of baking soda to create your own fabric freshener. This can help you save and create the scent that you like.

Mouthwash – you can use one or two drops of an essential oil mixed with honey and warm water for your mouth wash. The essential oils tea tree, peppermint, and cinnamon are suitable to use for mouthwash. Gargle the mouthwash for about 30 seconds and for best results, this can be repeated every four hours.

Mice Repellent – essential oils can repel mice from visiting or invading your home. Peppermint, for instance, proves to be an effective oil to deter mice invasion. Mix a few drops with water and put the solution in a spray bottle. Spray in areas where mice travel or hide.

Calm your dog- to prevent stress and anxiety (e.g. separation anxiety) of your dog, spray lavender oil solution a few inches above your dog's head. This will calm your pet. Exercise care and caution when there are pets other than your dog, e.g. cats, as they may not be able to tolerate the scent. Some oils are also not suitable for other pets.

Disinfectant – some oils, such as lemon oil, can disinfect your home. Spray lemon oil solution in the bathroom, sink, floor, and other areas prone to the presence of microbes.

Kill Mold – you can use one teaspoon of tea tree oil added to a cup of water for this. This can kill mold that can be found in areas of your home by simply sprinkling an amount of the mixture to the affected area and leaving it there. The essential oil tea tree is suitable for this purpose.

Vaporizers – you can use essential oils to clear bad odors in your home. Essential oils have antiseptic properties which can help kill bacteria and viruses in the air. This can also help stop the spread of infectious diseases in your home.

Hide Unpleasant Odors – you can use five to six drops of essential oils mixed with 1 cup of baking soda to remove unpleasant odors. This can be used in your home mats and carpets. Drop the mixture in small amounts around your mats and carpets and it will remove the unpleasant odors. Lavender and orange essential oils can be used for this purpose.

Natural Home Cleaner – you can use essential oil as a healthy substitute to chemical-based cleaners. These oils can remove difficult stains, freshen up your linens, and clean the air without toxic residues of chemical-based cleaners. Some of the best essential oils you can use for this purposes are the following: thieves, lemon, pine, lavender, orange, and cinnamon.

Chapter 5:

Natural Treatments Using Essential Oils

One way to save on cost of expensive treatments is to benefit from using essential oils. Here, you'll find four (4) ways to use essential oils as natural treatments you can do at home.

Skin Care

Sin care is an expensive treatment. Aside from the cost, chemical-based skin care products can be toxic to your body. This is especially true with long-term exposure to the products. The solution is to start substituting your usual cosmetic and skin care products with essential oils.

The following table illustrates how.

Usual Cosmetic & Skin Care Products	Essential Oil
Anti-aging	Apricot Kernel to hydrate skin Frankincense to reduce age spots Sweet Almond to protect the skin against harmful UV rays, prevent dryness, and maintain elasticity Geranium for cell regeneration Lemon oil to avoid wrinkles and fine lines Cypress lessens occurrence of varicose veins Argan oil to restore skin's elasticity

	Pomegranate Seed delays the aging process
	Neroli minimizes wrinkles and fine lines
	Sandalwood smoothens the skin
	Myrrh promotes younger-looking skin
	Carrot seed oil to protect skin from UV rays
	Rosemary tightens skin and prevents sagging
	Sea Buckthorn Berry reverses skin aging
Natural Remedy for Skin Disorders	Lemon works as anti-bacterial, anti-fungal, and anti-microbial that can help clear acne breakouts
	Cypress to reduce the appearance of varicose veins and to repair broken capillaries
	Tea Tree or Roman Chamomile for sunburns
	Peppermint to soothe irritated and itchy skin
	Clove or Peppermint and Grapefruit for corns
	Lavender, Geranium, or Frankincense for wrinkles
	Lavender to treat minor skin burns and rashes caused by diapers
	Oregano to treat callous and thick skin
	Myrrh heals cracked skin and is good for facial skin
	Chamomile and Lavender for diaper rash
	Thyme is best for dermatitis and eczema
	Rose and Frankincense to lighten scars
	Tea Tree and Oregano for fungal skin infections
	Geranium and Myrrh for skin bumps
	Geranium and lavender for dry and dehydrated skin

	Tea Tree and Peppermint to get rid of scabies
	Lavender and myrrh can reduce stretch marks and cure skin ulcers. When combined with geranium, these three oils are good for impetigo

See to it that when you use essential oils for skin care, you follow the safety guidelines. Always perform a skin test before you proceed with the regimen.

First Aid

Some essential oils can work as your first defense or first aid against pain or injury. Dr. Axe, a natural medicine expert and a certified nutrition specialist, recommends the following essential oils to form part of your first aid kit:

Essential Oil	First Aid For
Lavender	Minor cuts and wounds, minor burns, stings, rashes, scrapes, relieves stress and anxiety, promotes sleep following a trauma
Frankincense	Anti-inflammatory disease and disorders, reduces scarring, heals bruises, promotes healing and stops the bleeding of wounds, clears sinus congestion
Peppermint	Heals digestive disorders, reduces or relieves muscle and joint pain, help treat asthma and bronchitis, clears sinus congestion, drives away fever and headaches
Melaleuca	Works as anti-infection, filtrates and cleans the air of pathogens and allergens to stop and prevent airborne diseases,

Weight Loss

Treatments for losing weight are usually expensive. Often, you only get temporary results from such treatments. Here are three of the best essential oils that can reduce the cost of your weight loss. At the same time, these oils also promote long-term weight loss results.

Cinnamon

This essential oil helps in regulating your blood sugar. According to Dr. Oz, if you balance your blood sugar, you can keep off your excess weight. This will allow you to enjoy long-term weight loss results. Add to the weight loss is that cinnamon can help in the treatment of Type 2 diabetes mellitus. This oil also aids the other essential oils to promote weight loss.

Grapefruit

It contains a natural substance, d-limonene, that improves the production and functions of digestive enzymes. These enzymes are necessary for breaking down food particles into nutrients. The ability of your body to metabolize food into nutrients affects your weight significantly. If digestive enzymes are deficient, you will find it difficult to get rid of your excess weight.

Grapefruit also has properties that help in toning, overeating, and cellulite. Inhaling the diffused oil can help lower cravings and avoid overeating. A glass of water with drops of grapefruit essential oil can enhance the flavor of the water and help avoid overeating.

Peppermint

This essential oil can suppress unnecessary cravings for food. Controlling your appetite is one of the critical ways to lose weight. If you eat only to satisfy your real hunger, you can prevent unnecessary calories to enter your body. A part of the brain tells you when to feel full and peppermint has an effect on this part of the brain which makes it effective for controlling your appetite.

Peppermint oil is also effective in melting belly fat. This is crucial since belly fat is the most dangerous type of fat in the body. It can trigger cardiovascular diseases such as heart attack and stroke.

Hair Growth

If you have problems with your hair and scalp, then you'll find certain essential oils as an effective natural remedy. For instance, from Chapter 3, you have learned that Lavender essential oil is a proven remedy for alopecia areata, an autoimmune disease characterized by hair loss.

There are other oils like sage and rosemary essential oils that can promote the good condition of your scalp, stimulate hair growth, and/or thicken your hair. Here's how to do it:

1. Dilute the essential oil of your choice. Refer to the table of how to dilute essential oils in Chapter 2.
2. Pour a few drops of the diluted oil on your palm. Massage your scalp gently in circular motion with the oil.
3. For best results, do not rinse immediately. Cover your scalp with a hot towel for about 10-20 minutes.
4. Rinse your scalp. Follow with mild shampoo. Rinse thoroughly.

As the purity and quality of oil is critical in getting desirable results, it is important that you get your essential oils only from trusted sellers. Not all oils that you can find in the market are 100% pure and of high quality. As there are no standards for quality and purity, your best option is to verify the reputability of the seller.

Bonus Chapter:
Proper Storage of Essential Oils

One way to make sure essential oils remain safe for use is to know how to store them properly.

Storage conditions that the essential oils experience can affect their shelf life which determines when it is still good for use.

Proper storage is also important to keep essential oils from the reach of children and avoid accidents to happen. Here are some tips on how to store your essential oils properly.

Avoid Heat and Direct Sunlight

Keep your essential oils in a place where there is no direct sunlight. Avoid storing the oils in places near your window or wherever there is direct contact with sunlight.

Direct sunlight can cause a color change in an essential oil which can lead to changes in its therapeutic benefits.

Heat should also be avoided because essential oils are flammable. Essential oils can only tolerate a certain temperature of heat.

When exposed to heat above their maximum tolerable temperature, these essential oils will ignite.

Essential oils should be stored in a room with cool temperature and away from direct sunlight. These oils can also be stored inside the refrigerator with temperatures ranging from 5 to 10 degrees Celsius.

Use Bottles with Dark Shades

Essential oils should be stored in bottles with dark shades or colors. These kind of bottles are good to use when storing essential oils because they can filter out the UV rays from the sun.

Even when stored in bottles with dark shades or colors, the essential oils should still be stored away from direct sunlight.

Exposure in sunlight can accelerate the process of oxidation which can affect the therapeutic properties of the oil.

Avoid Exposure to Oxygen and Moisture

Exposure of an essential oil to oxygen will lead to the deterioration of the oil. Oxidation can also lead to the loss of therapeutic properties within the essential oil. This too can cause the essential oil to evaporate more quickly.

Moisture can cause the essential oil to be cloudy and can lead to deterioration of the oil. This too can damage the bottle of the essential oil.

Do Not Use Plastic Containers

Plastic containers are not suitable for essential oil storage since most essential oils can gradually destroy or melt the plastic material. High concentrated essential oils should not be stored in plastic containers.

Storage Boxes

If you do not have space in your refrigerator for your essential oils, using a special box just for these oils is advisable. Keeping your essential oils in these boxes can help you in organizing your stuff and also help keep away these oils from the reach of children.

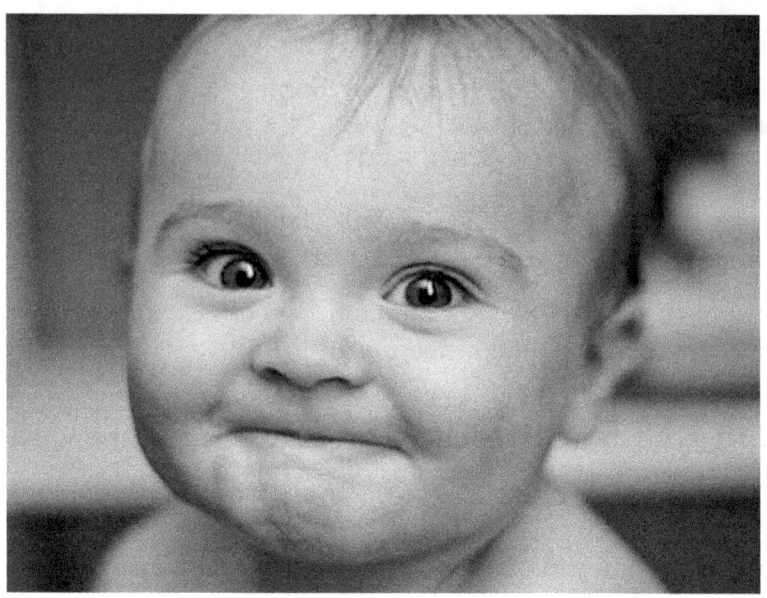

Conclusion

Thank you again for downloading this book!

I hope this book was able to help you get started in benefiting from essential oils. Discard prevailing myths as they will only prevent you from using essential oils successfully.

You have learned that not all oils are pure and of high quality. This is important and worth remembering because the therapeutic benefits can only be yours when you use pure and high quality essential oils.

Therefore, you must be careful in buying your essential oils. Chapter 2 has provided you with basic information on how to distinguish essential oils from fragrance oils.

It also presented you with information on how to determine purity and quality in the absence of standards.

Understand that not all essential oils have the same effect. Further, some oils are safer to use than the others. From Chapter 3, you have learned that three of the safer oils are lavender, chamomile, and lemon.

This does not mean, though, that you can forego safety precautions when using essential oils. You still need to exercise care and caution to prevent and avoid side effects.

Chapter 4 equipped you with basic information on how to use or apply essential oils. Two of the safer methods are: (1) aromatherapy, and (2) topical use.

While ingestion is another method to benefit from essential oils, you should only use this method upon the recommendation and guidance of your health expert. You've also learned from this chapter how to use the oils for your home.

When used properly, essential oils are effective natural remedy. In chapter 5, you've discovered ways to use the oils for natural treatments.

These treatments are economical, safer, and practical.

These are unlike most treatments using chemical-based products and ingredients which are not only costly, but also carry the risks of adverse effects due to toxic substances.

The next step is to put the discoveries and learnings from this book to good use. You, your family, your pet/s, and your home will surely benefit from essential oils when you apply what you have learned.

However, do not limit yourself to the information herein. Continue to explore, and you'll get to appreciate the value of essential oils more.

Finally, if you enjoyed this book, then I'd like to ask you for a favor, would you be kind enough to leave a review for this book on Amazon?

It'd be greatly appreciated.

Please leave a review for this book on Amazon!

Thank you and good luck!

www.ingramcontent.com/pod-product-compliance
Lightning Source LLC
Chambersburg PA
CBHW070450290526
45791CB00005B/2112